Eat Healthy, My Sweetie

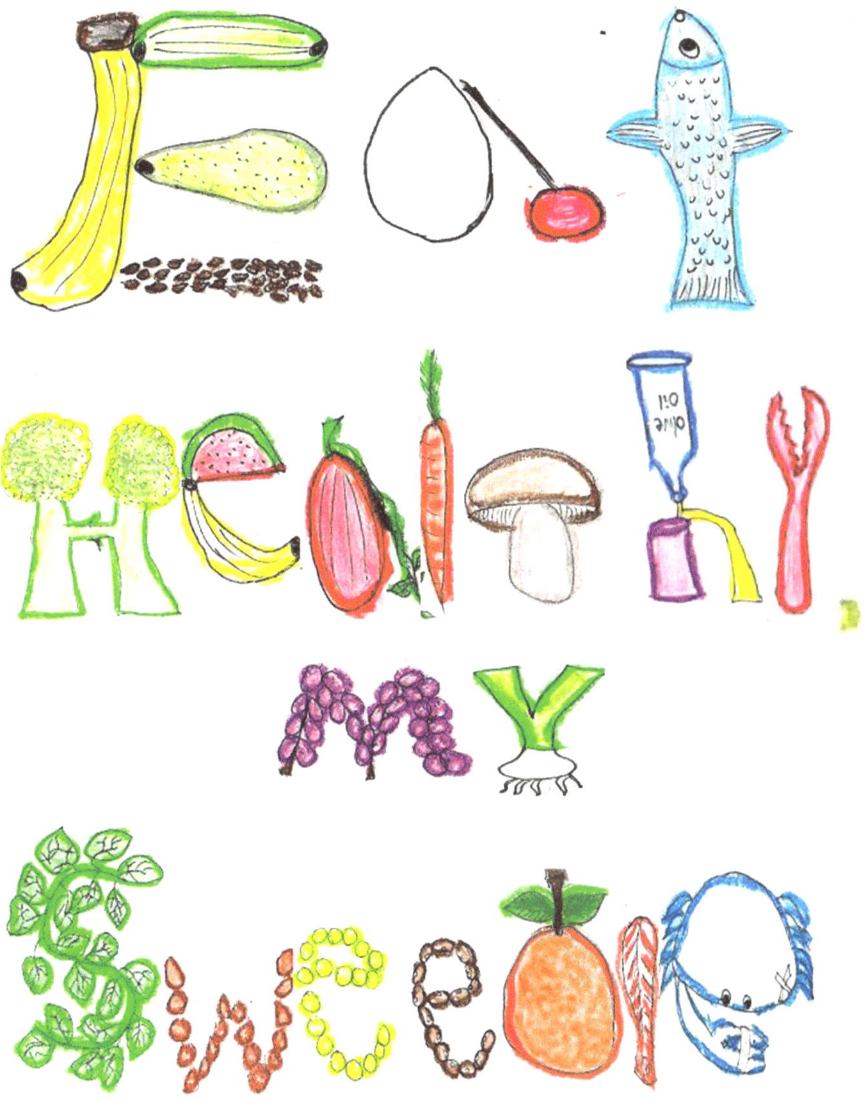

Written and Illustrated by

Tien Huang

Order this book online at www.trafford.com
or email orders@trafford.com

Most Trafford titles are also available at major online book retailers.

Printed in the United States of America.

ISBN: 978-1-4269-7448-9

Library of Congress Control Number: 2011910912

Trafford rev. 06/27/2011

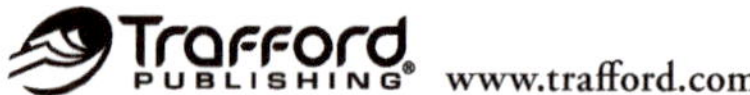

www.trafford.com

North America & international
toll-free: 1 888 232 4444 (USA & Canada)
phone: 250 383 6864 • fax: 812 355 4082

Eat Healthy, My Sweetie

Written and Illustrated by

Tien Huang

Thank you to all of my aficionados.

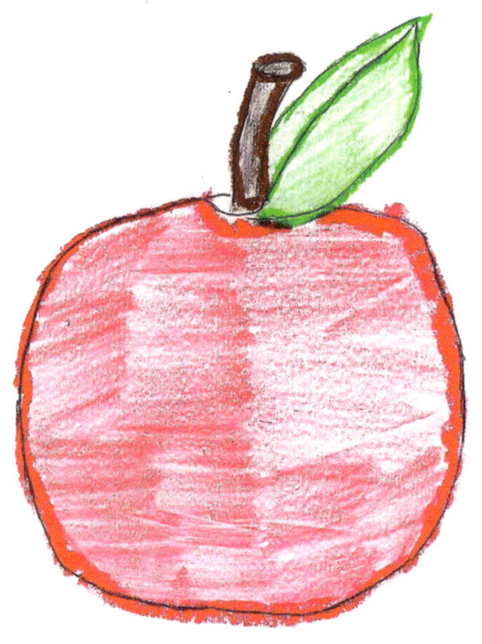

Come now sweetie, don't be a terror. Please just eat one red apple every morning. The antioxidants will keep your blood arteries healthy and you won't one day need to swallow bitter pills unnecessarily.

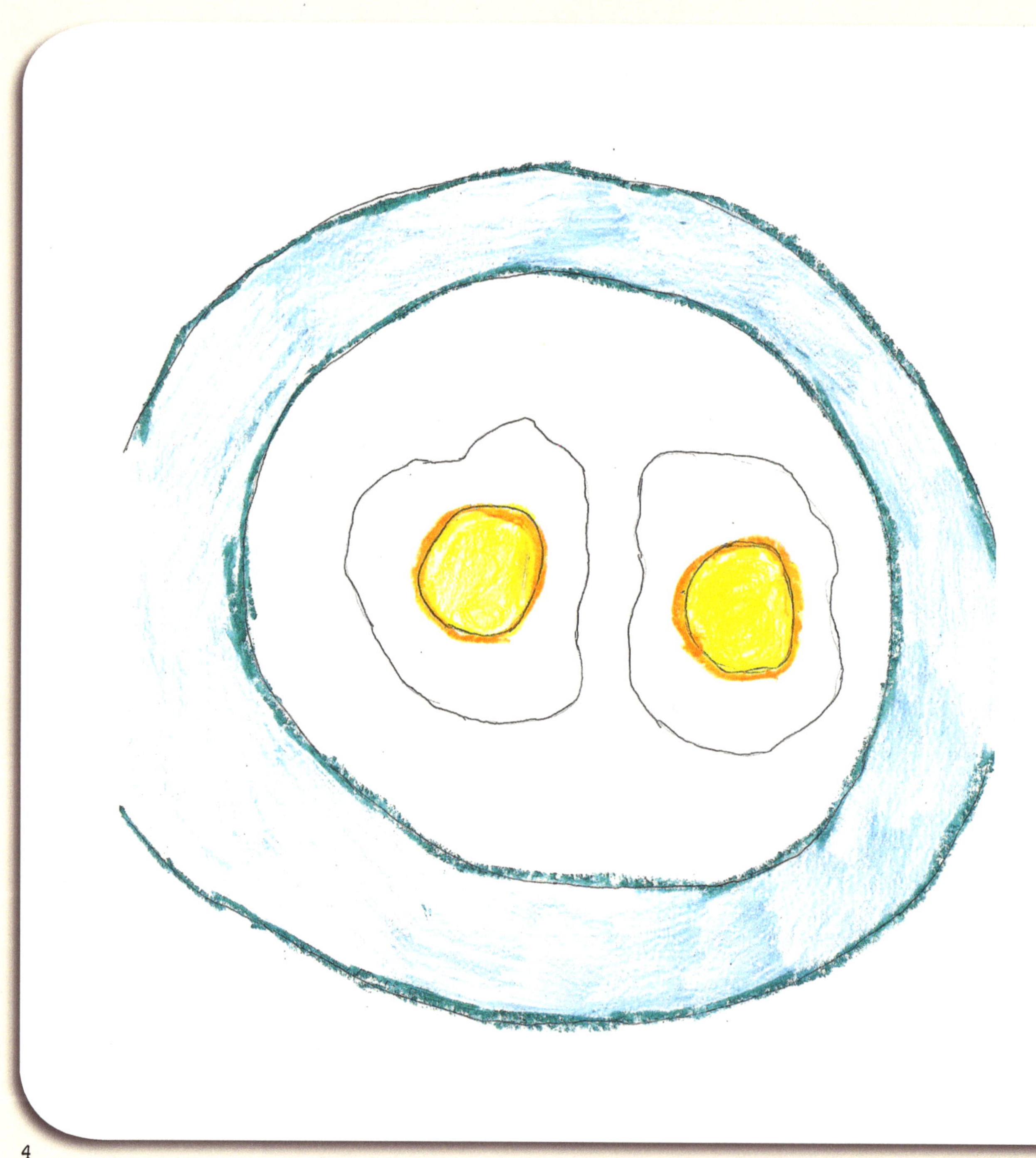

I promise you that two sunny-side-up fried eggs will make your mouth water. They provide protein, vitamins, and minerals to keep your body working. I admit, eggs have good and bad fats so eat your two eggs cautiously and you'll skip around happily.

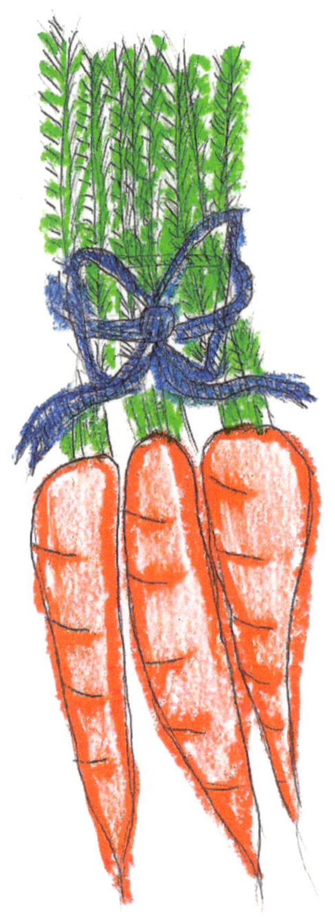

Three long stems of orange carrots call out your name as you reach out for a crunch. Come on, buddy! Crunch crunch crunch! Carrots taste sweet and juicy just like candy. Don't you want to see better at night, my sweetie?

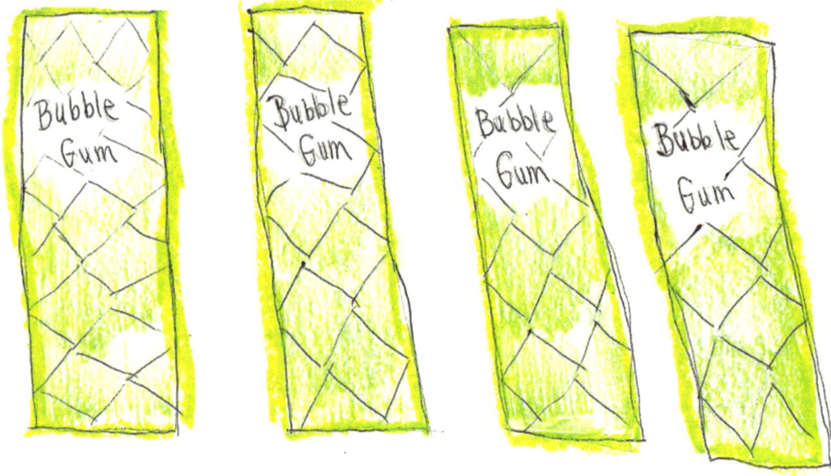
Bubble
Gum
Bubble
Gum
Bubble
Gum
Bubble
Gum

If you ever ask me for four pieces of sweet gum to chew on, I will say to you: "No, you can't have four pieces of soft, sweet, and chewy bubble gum to chew on! Do you want to live with painful cavities and no teeth for the rest of your life?"

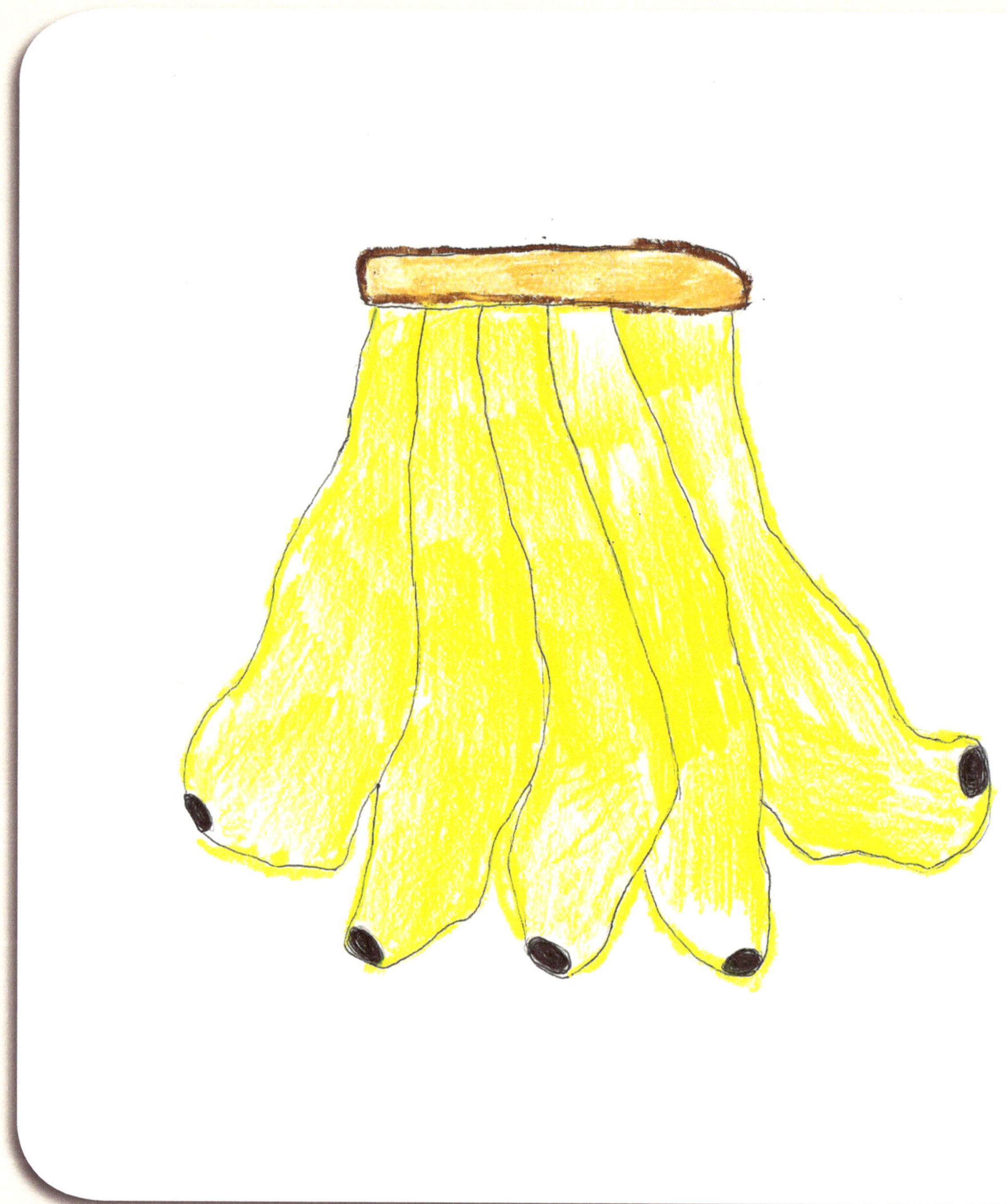

A bunch of five yellow bananas begs for you on the kitchen counter, my dear. I know you hate eating so many fruits. Please just know that the potassium in the banana will make you more alert so that when you put your hand on a hot stove one day, you'll quickly move it away and won't get burned very badly.

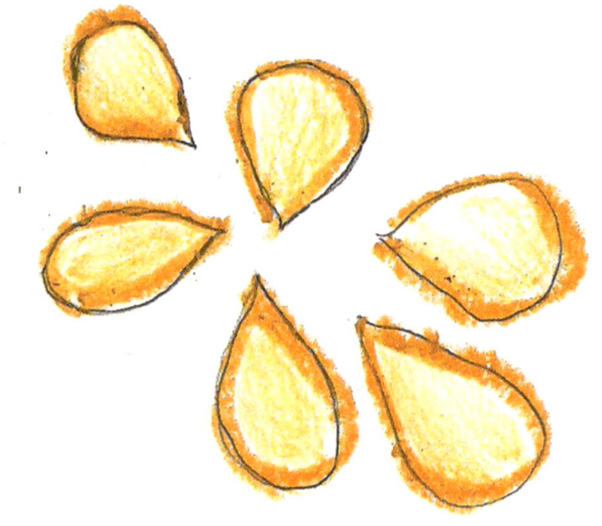

Every afternoon, six kernels of flaxseed will be fun to eat. You should really try to eat more than just six kernels though. The fiber in the flaxseed will help you digest your food so that you won't have a painful, hard time on the potty.

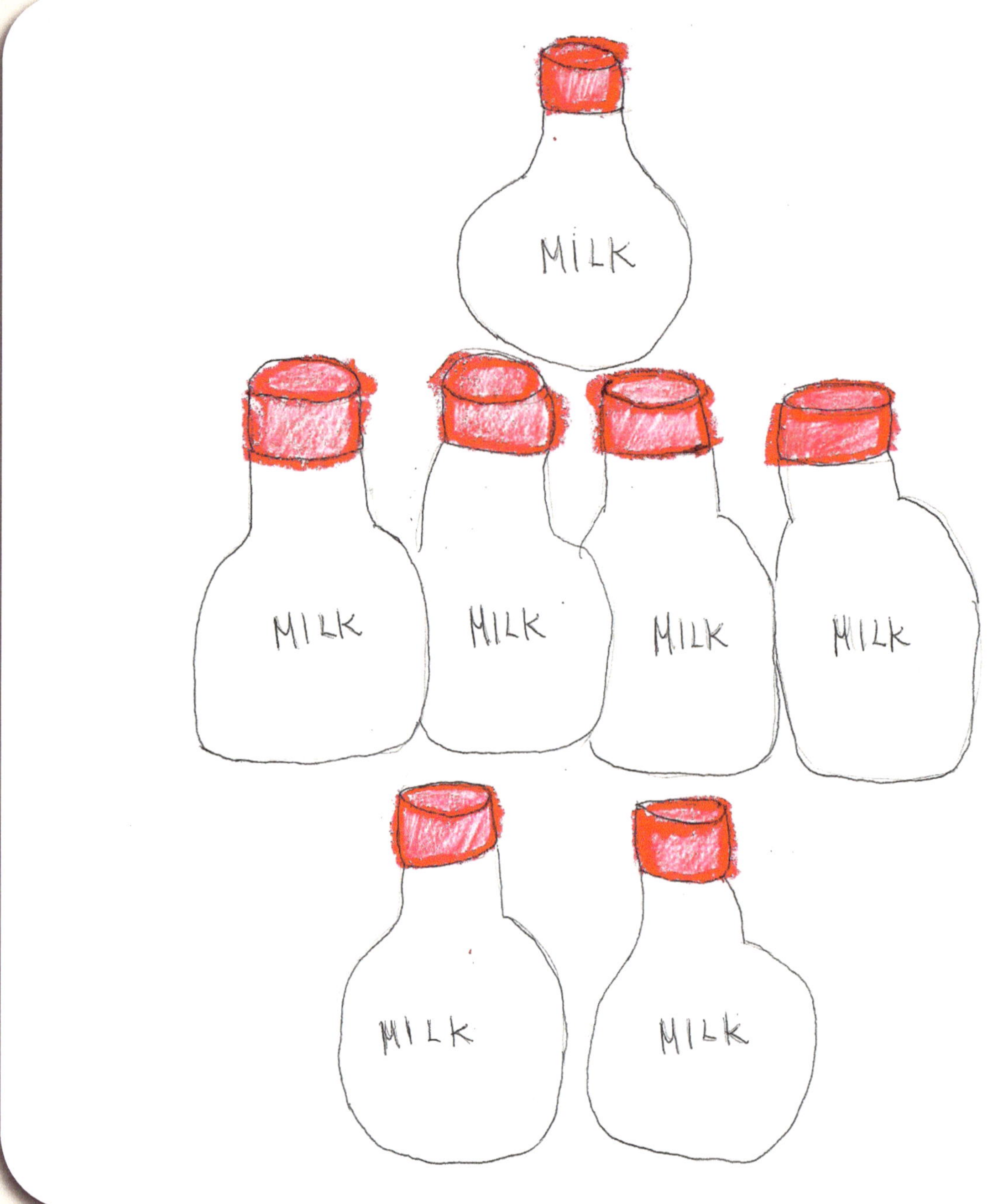
MILK
MILK
MILK
MILK
MILK
MILK
MILK

Seven pints of milk sit in the refrigerator. Come on, my prodigy, you know the calcium in the white liquid will make your teeth and bones hard and mighty! Drink a pint with some whole grain cereal or drink a pint alone like water to keep you cool from the hot sun!

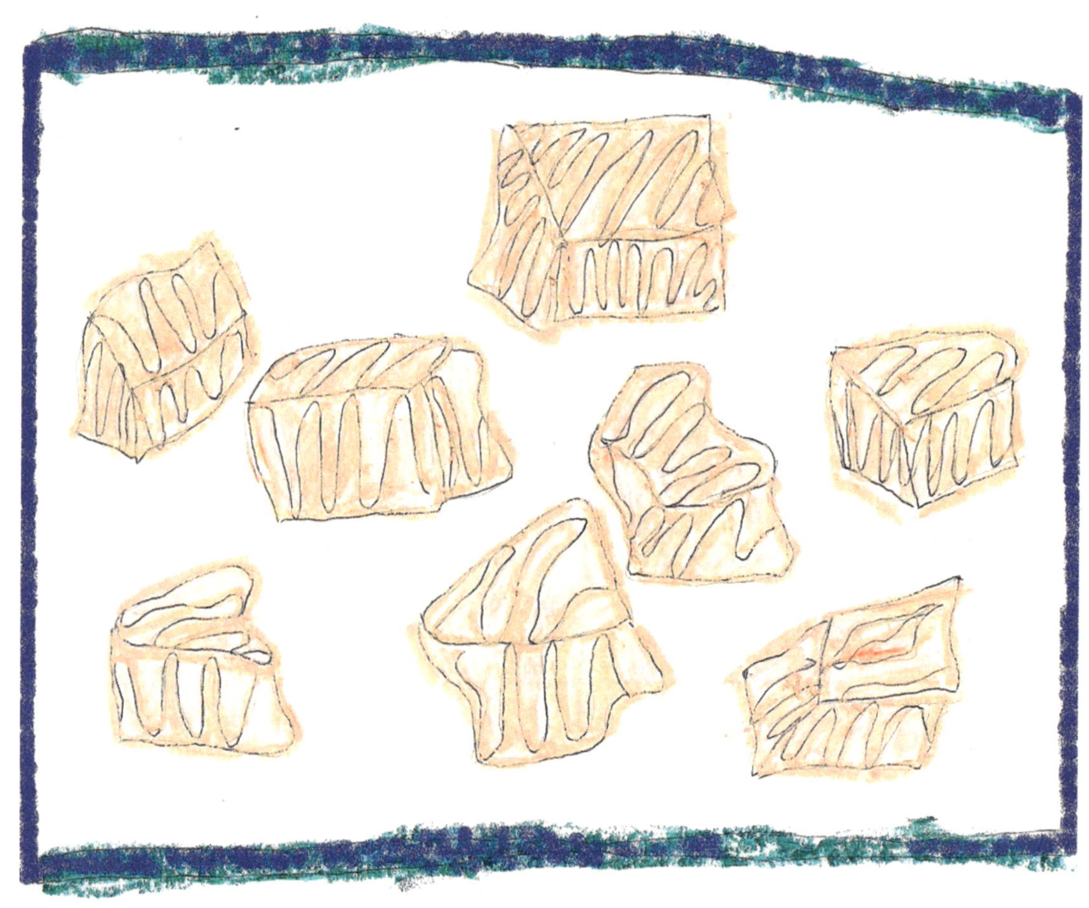

Eight small pieces of salmon sit in the refrigerator waiting for you to eat for dinner. Is the smell of fish so bad that you just won't even look at it, my picky eater? You're missing out on Omega-3 good fats in the fish meat that can prevent you from dying prematurely.

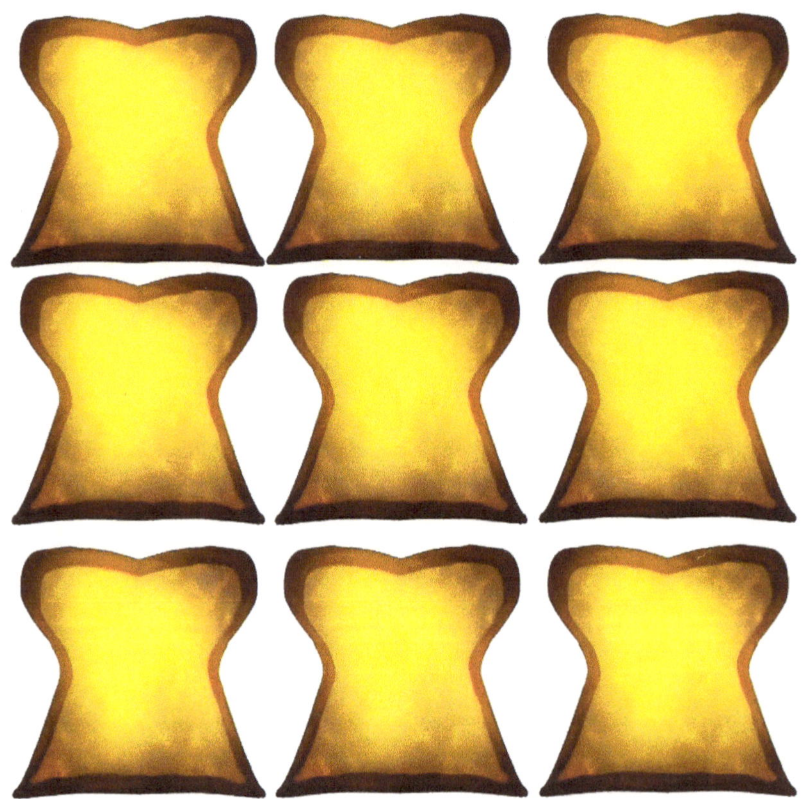

Nine slices of whole wheat bread sit on the dinner table every night. I made them just for you. You know you like eating fresh, warm, and toasty bread that won't cause you to turn chubby. Why won't you take just one slice to thank me for my efforts?

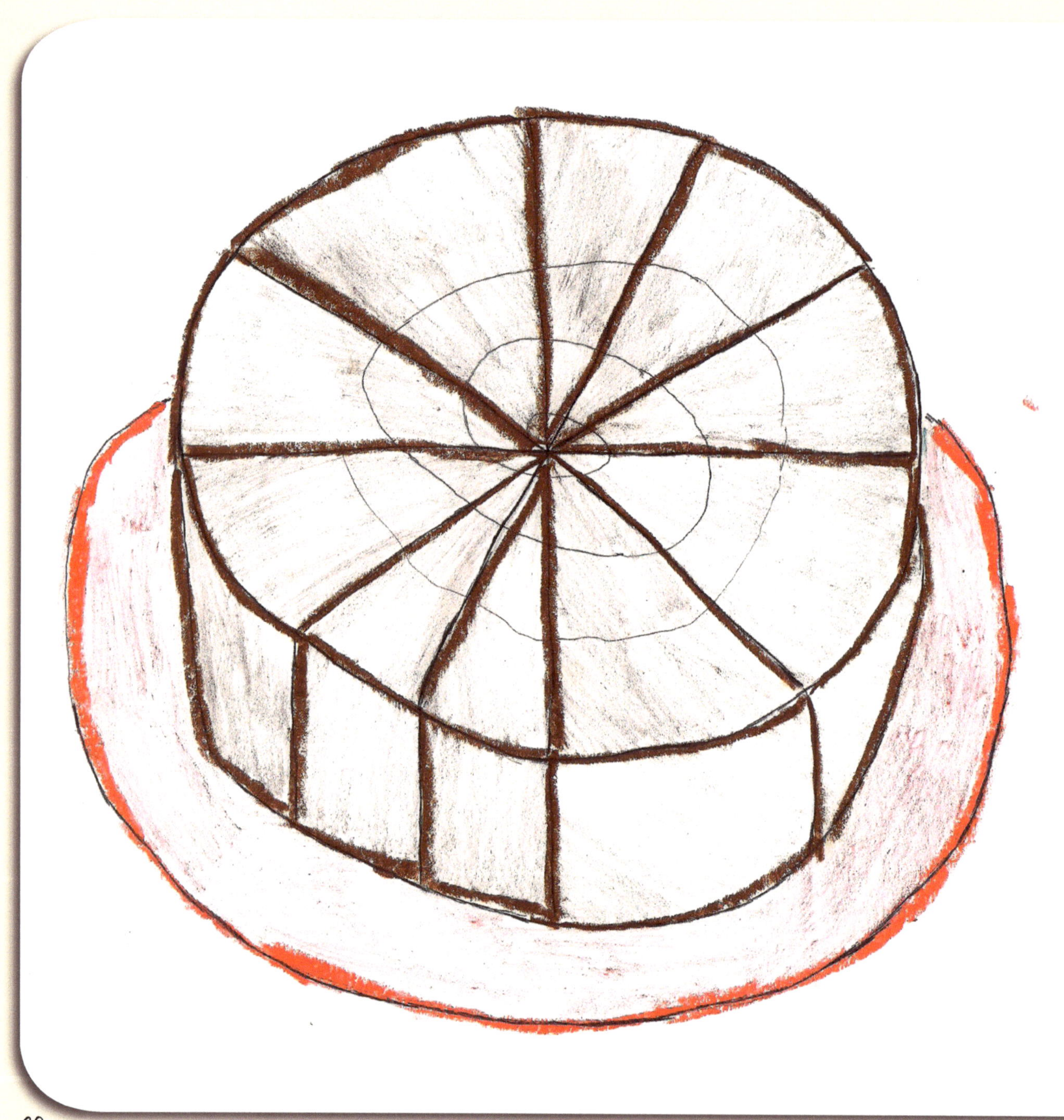

A whole chocolate fudge cake cut into ten slices sits waiting on the table too. Your majesty, don't be tempted to nibble a bite from the smallest slice because you haven't yet cheated on your diet.

Off to bed you go! Count some sheep in your sleep without nibbling or looking back at the moist, sweet cake my beautiful angel.

www.ingramcontent.com/pod-product-compliance
Lightning Source LLC
LaVergne TN
LVHW070208110826
845147LV00002B/531

* 9 7 8 1 4 2 6 9 7 4 4 8 9 *